Beginner's Guide to Bodybuilding
By Jeff Haney

Table of Contents

Introduction

Before I begin, I would like to point out that this book is targeted majorly towards lifters that are just starting out. There is a lot of information here for those of you with more experience also, however it will be less useful for anyone with a few years of training already under your belt.

With that out of the way, this guide will be a massive aid if you are looking to get into the sport of bodybuilding or even if you are just trying to find the edge you need to break some PRs in the gym. Over the years I have had to go through a large amount of trial and error to truly understand how my body works and what works in the gym. I have read books, searched the web, consulted my local gym rats, anything I needed to be most efficient with my time spent training. The problem with this is that there was not really any one place that I could go to for a collection of information that actually mattered. I would spend hours researching a single topic just to find one bit of relevant information to what I wanted to know, and the entire time all I could think was how badly I wished there was a single book or website I could go to that would explain everything I had questions about without the extra fluff or jargon that I did not understand.

Now that I have finally reached a level of understanding that I am satisfied with, I decided I would fill the void and provide everyone with a solid reference to begin training without wasting any time. Since this is a guide for beginners, I will not cover the topics of posing or competitions; this is strictly a book about getting your body in peak condition. I will also avoid discussing a few things that I do not believe are necessary for beginners to worry about until being at least several years into training correctly.

I would advise anyone completely new to the gym scene to begin by skipping ahead to the "Common Terms" section of the book and briefly read through the words there. Most are not overly complicated however it would be a good idea to have a general understanding of the terms so that you know what is being discussed over the course of this text. If there is anything mentioned in the book that you do not understand such as a specific workout or supplement, head to the section "Additional Resources" and I am sure that you will find ample information on anything you need.

Finally, one more important thing to note before delving into this book: bodybuilding requires dedication. Forget all of the "Get ripped in six days!" and "Gain 50 pounds of muscle in a month!" lines you have been fed. This simply does not happen similar to the fact that you will not become a millionaire in a week despite what many internet ads would leave you to believe. That being said, it is entirely possible and in fact guaranteed that you will progress far beyond where you are now physically if you stay committed to your training and follow all of the suggestions mentioned in this book. That is right, all of them. If you are expecting to get give it your all in the gym but have a poorly controlled diet then you are likely to get overall poor results relative to if you take all factors into account. If you are prepared to make the commitment and transform your body, read on.

Diet

First things first, diet. This is the single most overlooked aspect of bodybuilding hands down, and yet it is also the most important. The reason most people avoid following a correct diet is because it is more restrictive on their personal lives than training. You can have a workout regardless of what is going on aside from time constraints, however if you are on a diet then you might be forced to resist the second slice of pizza or going out for beers with friends. This is simply a sacrifice you have to make if you are going to get the most out of your body.

Contrary to popular belief, though, dieting is not nearly as bad as you might suspect. It is not all crazy low carb diets or meals entirely of vegetables (though that is an option). Instead you can follow the IIFYM rule, which stands for If It Fits Your Macros. Basically this just means that anything is fair game as long as it does not go too far over or under your macro limit for the day. But before figuring out what your macros will be for the day, you must determine whether you are bulking or cutting.

Bulking vs. Cutting

Most people believe that a diet is a way to eat to lose weight. This is incorrect. A diet can more correctly be defined as a predefined eating habit or schedule with the purpose of reaching a certain goal. This goal can be to lose weight, gain muscle, or any number of things. At this point food becomes a tool used to further your body rather than simply a snack.

Along with the fact that a diet is not limited to being a way to lose weight, you should also understand that many people concerned with their weight have no intention of losing it but rather gaining it. These are usually people known as "hard-gainers", someone who is below average weight that would like to pack on pounds and muscle. Once you decide whether your goal is mainly to lose weight or gain muscle, you can decide whether you are bulking or cutting.

Bulking is exactly how it sounds, a way of increasing your weight and adding muscle mass. If you are a hard-gainer then your first step in the world of bodybuilding is to bulk. The specifics will be detailed in the next few sections, but what it generally means is that you will be eating more and doing a bit less cardio than if you what cutting. The opposite of this means that if you would like to begin the path to losing weight, in general you will be eating less and doing a significant amount of cardio than if you were bulking.

After the initial phase of the first few months when you become relatively content with your body you will likely want to start joining into the loosely structured bulking and cutting seasons. Put simply, bulking season is during the winter months when you will pack on muscle mass and you will begin cutting shortly prior to summer in order to better show off your progress.

Weight Gain/Loss

If weight gain or weight loss is your primary goal and you are unconcerned with aesthetics (how your body/muscles look), there are several things that might be useful to remember. First, when you first begin weight training it is likely that you will pack on a few extra pounds even if you are cutting. The reason for this is that muscle weighs more than fat so even if visibly you will appear skinnier you might still gain as far as the scale is concerned. The other is the fact that weight is not concerned with what you are eating, simply how much. What I mean is that to gain a pound you must consume 3500 additional calories than you burn. To lose a pound, you must consume 3500 less calories. A good way to apply this information is the 500 calories per day method (by adjusting your calorie intake by 500 per day, you can gain or lose about a pound per week depending on your goals). There is no set number for how many calories an individual burns in a day, so use trial and error to find out your maintenance limit. If you are trying to gain weight slowly add a hundred calories a week. If you gained less than a pound that week, increase your daily limit. If you gained more than a pound then you will decrease your daily limit. The same concept would be applied when trying to lose weight. Remember that you should not be gaining or losing much more than a pound per week as this means you are in too much of a calorie surplus or deficit.

Maintenance

To understand how many calories you should consume to maintain you weight, follow these guidelines: eat 1 gram of protein per pound of bodyweight, eat 1.5 grams of carbs per pound of bodyweight, and eat 1 gram of fats per 4 pounds of bodyweight per day. When you are cutting, lower your carb intake by about 90 grams and your protein intake by about 10. By contrast if your goal is to bulk up you will want to increase your protein consumption by 50 grams per day and your fats by 30.

Carbs

Carbs, possibly one of the most hated words among fad diets. The reason for this is that carbs are basically used up as energy during day to day activities. If there are less carbs available, the body will use stored fat as energy instead thus causing you to lose body fat. Lower carbs while cutting is effective, however you cannot completely cut them out as this is dangerous and unhealthy. There are two types of carbs: simple and complex. Simple carbs are sugar, found in fruits and junk food. Complex carbs are found in rice and pasta. The function difference between the two is that simple carbs are digested more quickly which causes them to more easily turn into fat if they are not used as energy soon. Complex carbs on the other hand get used slowly over a longer period of time and are more likely to be used up efficiently as energy to power your body. For this reason you should try to get most of your carbs from complex sources rather than simple sugars.

Note: This is a simplified explanation, but that is all you really need to know as a beginner.

Protein

Protein is regarded as the most important nutrient of all by bodybuilders, and for good reason. Protein is the building block of muscles. As with everything in this guide you can be incredibly detailed and thorough in a discussion about proteins, but we will stick with the basics for the purposes of this book. Just keep in mind that proteins come in many shapes and sizes based on the source that you get them from and these different types of protein will be utilized over a varying range of times.

Basically, you will get your protein from two different sources: food and supplements. For the most effective use of these proteins, you should consume them spread throughout the day and not all during a single meal. It is best to get most of your protein from food, but not just any food. If you want the greatest benefit you should try to get it from varying sources including: beef, poultry, fish, milk, eggs, and nuts. A prime example of a bodybuilder's meal is chicken breast (protein) and white rice (carbs). You do not need anything fancy to get a nutritious meal. If you cannot get your macros for the day, supplements can help fill the gap and that is where protein powder comes in. But more on that later.

Although I do not want to get too deep into this subject, different proteins from different foods will be utilized at different times by your body. This is similar to the concept covered previously about how simple carbs are processed faster than complex carbs. For the most part, protein from foods are in the medium time range and you do not need to worry too much about it, just make your meals try to hit your macro limit. This is different from protein supplements. Protein powder primarily comes in two forms: whey (fast release) and casein (slow release). Just keep this in mind for now and I will return to it in a bit.

Fats

Many people consider fat to be a bad thing, whether dieting or not fat is just assumed to be bad in any context, but this is not actually correct. There are many cases when fat is very helpful and at times even essential.

The first case where fats are beneficial is if you plan on bulking. As discussed previously, gaining weight is a matter of calories consumed versus calories burned. A single gram of either protein or carbs is 4 calories, while a single gram of fat is 9 calories. You can see how this can quickly help if you are a hard-gainer looking to pack on some extra pounds. This also makes reaching your daily calorie intake a little easier if you are on a budget.

Another reason that fats should be considered important is the term "fat-soluble". This refers to nutrients that cannot be absorbed by the body unless in the presence of fat. Some of these nutrients are vitamin A, vitamin D, vitamin E and vitamin K. Without fat these would be unable to be taken in thus making them useless to your body.

While these two attributes definitely are desirable, fat has not gotten a bad reputation for no reason. As there are good fats, there are also bad fats. It is important to try to take in mainly beneficial fats and avoid those that will harm you. Saturated fats and trans fats are in the "bad" category, as these are known to raise cholesterol and generally lower overall health. Opposite of that is monounsaturated, polyunsaturated, and Omega-3 (chemically classed as a polyunsaturated fat). Monounsaturated fats are mainly found in natural foods like nuts, avocados, olive oil, and grape-seed oil, corn oil and canola oil. Both it and the polyunsaturated fats, which can be found in vegetable oils, sunflower and cottonseed oil, are proven to increase cardiovascular health. Omega-3 fats are generally categorized separately from polyunsaturated fats and have a myriad of health benefits such as helping to prevent cancer growth and improving brain function. These can be found in many types of fish as well as walnuts. As with all things, fats are only as good or bad as you make them. Take the time to read labels and consume the favorable fats and you will find they are just another tool to further your body and your experience in the gym.

Water

It has undoubtedly been drilled into your mind time and time again that water is important. Water is one of the most vital components of life as well as in bodybuilding. Although almost everyone knows that water is important, not everyone knows why. Here are a few reasons that are relevant to you as a bodybuilder.

One of the most obvious benefits is that consuming water prevents dehydration. During a workout your muscles heat up which causes sweating and water loss. Having a sufficient amount of water in your system can prevent the negative effects of becoming dehydrated. Back and joint pain is one such drawback, which can be alleviated with an increase in water intake. Water also helps to cleanse your system by diluting acids.

Aside from these general advantages, water is even more essential when you are a dedicated lifter. Regular consumption will aid in digesting, transporting, and utilizing vital nutrients that function to build and repair muscle. In addition drinking a glass of cold water every now and then will restart the digestion function and use energy and burn calories as the water will first have to be heated to be used in other body functions.

Finally, there is a common misconception about water retention. Taking in a large amount of water is actually helpful in reducing water retention. Many people believe that the extra water weight on their body is caused by an excessive of water taken in and that less water will help them drop the weight, however this is opposite from the truth. Think of how a camel stores water in its hump. This is essentially what your body does if you take in an insufficient amount of fluids, it will store the water it does get in the event that you have to go a long time without water. To flush out water retention all that you have to do is drink more water.

It is debatable as to how much water is the right amount for a person, however among the bodybuilding community it is generally agreed that about a gallon a day is sufficient for an adult male (about 180 pounds). You can adjust this slightly to meet your needs, and remember that some foods as well as juices and milk include water in them as well. Whatever your preferred method, just find a way to stay amply hydrated throughout each day.

Meal Prep

If you have been following along, you will have noticed by now that keeping up a good diet is a time consuming task. If you factor in time needed for shopping for groceries, cooking, and eating you can easily see why dieting is often neglected. However, there is a way around this. The key to successfully sustaining a diet is time management. To cut down on shopping costs, buy anything that will not expire soon in bulk to reduce trips to the store. Take a similar approach with cooking. Select a day out of the week that you are not very busy and cook meals for the entire week and keep them stored. Each day you will already have the meal prepared and you will not need to waste time cooking. Doing this will save a considerable amount of time and effort.

You should also always try to spread out your meals throughout the entire day. Instead of eating 2 or 3 big meals a day, try to eat 4 or 5 smaller meals. This will help keep your metabolism active as well as help your body utilize all of the nutrients you take in. Finding the best time to eat is entirely dependent on your own personal schedule, however you should do your best to prioritize a meal first thing in the morning as well as a meal close to bedtime. The reason for this is that after waking up your body has been without food for the entire duration that you have been asleep. Eating right away helps get the nutrients into your body to fuel it for the day. This is the same reason why it is a good idea to eat close to the time you go to bed, leaving your body with food to digest during the night helps to minimize the time it will have to go without sustenance.

Supplements

A word of caution before I begin this section. Notice that all of the products located here are placed in the category of "supplements". The word "supplements" is key here, these are tools to be used to *supplement* your diet and training, not to replace it. It should also be made clear that not all supplements work as intended for every single person. Each person reading this has a different body and will likely react slightly different to each of these products. For the sake of steering you away from scam products, I will recommend what I personally use or have used in each of these categories. There are far too many different types of supplements to cover in a beginner's book, and most of it would not be easily understood by beginners anyway. Instead I will cover what I believe should be a staple in any serious lifter's supplement stack and do my best to help you understand what it is actually doing for you so you can decide whether you would like to invest in it or not.

Protein Powder

It is highly unlikely that anyone reading this has not heard of a protein shake before. If you have, you have likely asked the questions "When is the best time to drink a protein shake?" or "How much protein should I consume in a shake?" and the answers to these questions will vary based on the individual asking.

To answer "When is the best time to drink a protein shake?" you should remember that there are two main forms of protein powder: whey and casein. Whey is useful when you need the protein in your body quickly, such as first thing in the morning or immediately after a workout. This helps to replenish your body of nutrients lost while sleeping or after a hard workout. Casein does the exact opposite and is slowly digested. Slow absorption is good just before going to bed or during any part of the day when you will not be able to eat for an extended period of time.

As to "How much protein should I consume in a shake?" it depends on your current diet. Protein shakes are primarily used to fill a gap in a weight lifters macro limit for the day. For example, if you are short about 30 grams of protein for the day then one serving of casein (most protein powders give you around 25 grams of protein per serving) before bed mixed with a cup of milk can get you to your desired macro limit. It is fairly common to ensure that at least some of your protein comes from a whey protein shake immediately after a workout to restore your depleted nutrients, as this improves recovery time and muscle gains.

Although protein powder can be a great tool, be careful not to use it. The majority of protein and all nutrients for that matter should ideally come from your diet. My personal brand for protein supplements is Optimum Nutrition. You will see in a second that I go to them for most of my supplements, and for good reason. The products are high quality, good price, and I have never had an issue with customer service.

Pre-Workout

This is a broad category that varies greatly from product to product, but all pre-workouts have the same purpose: to push your workout as far as possible. Whether it is designed to increase your pump (the enlarged feeling your muscles get while exercising) or to improve your focus, pre-workout helps you go the extra mile. Although it can be a great benefit to your training regimen, you should be cautious of when you take it. Pre-workouts typically contain stimulants in them that will raise your heart rate, which means that taking them before a cardio session could potentially be dangerous. It will also be ineffective if you take it too early or too soon before a workout, make sure you read the directions for your specific product and follow them as closely as possible for the best results.

If you continue taking a single pre-workout over a long period of time, it is likely that your body will become increasingly tolerant to it. This will mean that to achieve the same results you will have to increase the dosage. Increasing the dosage past a certain point is not advised as it can be harmful to your health as well as put a dent in your wallet due to going through the supplement faster. One solution is to buy several different types of pre-workout with different formulas and alternate which one you take. Doing this will minimize the amount of tolerance that your body builds up and also give you the chance to use different pre-workouts suited to different days in the gym.

It has gotten to the point where I personally dislike going to the gym without taking some form of pre-workout. Not due to building up a dependency, just because I get so much more out of a session when I am focused and motivated. This might be a placebo effect but I find workouts much more effective after taking pre-workout. Although they do wonders for me, I personally have only responded to a few of the formulas that I have tried. From what I hear, pre-workout preference can vary drastically from person to person.

At the moment I am using Craze (from Driven Sports) and C4 (from Cellucor). These are what I have found to work for me, but I suggest trying samples of other formulas to figure out what works for you. Thankfully more supplements in this category are not too expensive given how helpful they are so shop around and find which ones you like and try to keep several different ones on hand to avoid building up a tolerance.

Creatine

This might be another supplement buzzword that you recognize, though anyone uneducated about creatine will insist that it is a steroid-like supplement and should be avoided at all costs. I cannot emphasize enough how wrong this is. Almost all serious lifters take creatine and it is by no means a steroid. What creatine does is supply your body with more ATP, the substance that fuels your muscles during a workout. Having more of this energy leads to being able to push out a few extra reps which in turn increases muscle growth. Creatine does not affect hormone levels which means it is not even remotely related to a steroid.

One complaint about creatine is that is in ineffective or harmful to your kidneys, however these complaints are invalid if you follow the directions carefully. On every container of creatine you are instructed to drink an appropriate amount of water with it, and if you follow these directions then it is not harmful in the slightest and it will produce the desired results.

There is a lot of controversy about when is the best time to take creatine. Some say it is best to take pre-workout, some say post-workout, and still others say that anytime during the day is fine. I personally have found that I get the intended effects regardless when I take it during the day, but find what best works for you.

Generally It is good to take a dosage of about 5 grams per day, however many people like to load when first starting to take creatine. What this means is to take about 10 grams for the first week or so to get the creatine into your system faster and thus get the benefits sooner. After this loading period you can return to 5 grams per day. Many companies also advise that you use it for a period of 12 weeks then discontinue for a period of 4 weeks (and repeat) so that your body does not begin to lower its own natural production of creatine.

There are many different forms of creatine, but for the most part they all perform the same function. Creatine monohydrate and creatine kre-alkalyn are the common ones mentioned among bodybuilders and there are a few differences but as a beginner either is fine. There has not been enough study to tell if the differences matter, but for reference creatine monohydrate has been used for a much longer time than kre-alkalyn and thus already has a reputation for effective use. I am currently using Optimum Nutrition's Micronized Creatine Powder, though for this specific supplement it is said that brand does not matter quite as much as it does for other supplements. As always, shop around and find what works best with your body.

Multi-Vitamins

"Pop a multi and lift" is possibly the best advice for a beginning weight lifter. Once your diet is in order, if you had to choose a single supplement to take I would advise that you go with a multi-vitamin. The benefits are severely underrated due to not being marketed as a bodybuilding supplement but the truth is that most people have some sort of vitamin or mineral deficiency. If you are one of these people, the simple lack of proper nutrients can hold back your lifting career far more than you think. Having a well-rounded diet will help but It is likely that you still will not be getting everything you need from food alone.

The effects and benefits are varied but just trust me when I say it only does good things. To name a few, a multi-vitamin will increase your overall energy levels, recovery time, bone strength, joint health, as well as many other things. However to get these effects you should be sure that you are taking the correct multi-vitamin (a Flintstone's chewable will not cut it). Make sure that what you are getting is labeled as some type of adult one-a-day. My personal vitamin of choice is Opti-Men by Optimum Nutrition. It comes at a great value and provides me with everything I need in a multi.

Bodybuilding vs. Powerlifting

One of the major mistakes that many people make is assuming that powerlifting and bodybuilding is the same thing. Both sports involve weight training and honestly that is about where the similarities end. This can be a problem if you are a potential powerlifter and you decide to follow the advice of a bodybuilder. The overall goal of a bodybuilder is to become as aesthetic (visually appealing) as possible, while a powerlifter's focus is solely on strength. Although you will become stronger through bodybuilding that is not your purpose in the same way that a powerlifter is not lifting for the purpose of getting more aesthetic.

Once you understand these differences you will be able to understand why you should train with your goal in mind. Generally, powerlifters will use higher weights in their exercises and perform fewer reps per set. An example is that a typical bodybuilder will perform an exercise doing 3 sets of 10 reps of a lower weight and a typical powerlifter will do the same exercise using a higher weight and performing 5 sets of 5 reps. This difference is due to the fact that muscles hypertrophy (increase in size) more easily at higher rep ranges. Using higher weights (and thus lower reps) will cause your muscles to grow stronger in order to better handle the heavier weight next time.

You will also notice that bodybuilders perform many more isolation exercises than powerlifters. Powerlifters primarily work the compound lifts (bench press, squat, deadlift) due to the fact that these are the lifts performed in competitions because of the sheer amount of weight that can be lifted with them. Bodybuilders on the other hand work to make their entire body symmetrical and their muscles as big as possible. When one muscle looks smaller in comparison to other muscles, a bodybuilder will take time to work that muscle harder to achieve a higher level of symmetry.

Perhaps the most glaring difference is the change in dieting between the two sports. While bodybuilders are encouraged to cut anytime fat becomes overly visible, there is not as much reason for a powerlifter to do so. With bulking comes an increase in strength, which leads to most powerlifters bulking endlessly for maximum gains in their lifts. The end result of this, of course, is that they are not as defined or as aesthetic as a bodybuilder. If your main goal is strength then I would suggest looking specifically for a powerlifter's training regimen and dieting habits. You will definitely gain strength through bodybuilding however you can become significantly stronger if that is your sole purpose for weight lifting.

Equipment
Free Weights vs. Machines

If you walk into the weight room of a gym chances are that you will see a section of free weights and a section of machines. This division is not simply because they operate differently but also because they exercise your muscles differently. To understand the difference you should first know what the two categories are composed of. Free weights are weights that you can pick up and move and all of the force used to perform the exercise comes from your body. These include dumbbells, barbells, kettlebells, etc. Machines are stationary devices that use a system of pulleys as well as your body to achieve the desired motion.

The main difference between the two is the mechanical assistance you receive from the machines while you receive no assistance with free weights. Since you can perform a similar movement with free weights as you can with a machine, where does the additional strength come from when using free weights? The answer is stabilizer muscles. These are smaller, supporting muscles that function the same way that pulleys do in machines to allow you to complete the motion of the exercise. What this means for your muscles is a more complete workout when using free weights as opposed to a machine.

For this reason most bodybuilders will primarily use free weights throughout their workout, but this does not mean machines are useless. Due to the fact that stabilizer muscles are not needed when using a machine they are good for isolating a specific muscle. For example, a bench press and a chest press are essentially the same motion. While a bench press mainly works your chest, it also receives support from your shoulders and triceps and smaller muscles to complete the motion. By contrast, the chest press machine relies on your chest alone and very little help from other muscles to complete the motion.

Machines might also be helpful if you need an extra exercise to fit into your workout or if all of the free weights are currently being used and you do not want to stall your workout. Aside from these times, I believe it is helpful for someone who has never trained before to start out for a week or two using machines and then moving on to free weights. This is a personal belief of mine but I think it helps to allow the muscles to be conditioned before starting a more intensive exercise.

Accessories

There are many items that can fit into this category but I am only going to touch on a few that I have personally tried. Accessories include lifting gloves, weight belts, straps, and other items that can help you while training in various ways.

Gloves and straps are intended to help you grasp the weight you are using better. Gloves directly increase your grip and can help for heavier lifts such as bench press and squats. Lifting chalk can be used for the same purpose and is generally preferred by most bodybuilders, but it must be reapplied each training session. Straps wrap around the weight and connect to your wrist to redistribute some of the weight and help make it easier to hold.

Weight belts are used during dips or pull-ups. These belts allow you to attach a weight to increase the difficult of the exercise once you progress past your body weight.

Squat belts help to stabilize your core while doing squats. This aids you in keeping yourself straight so that your form does not suffer and more energy can be spent working your legs.

Training

General Advice

Training is the first thing that anyone thinks of when they think of bodybuilding, even if diet and sleep are just as important. Even though the important of exercising is so clear many people still do not understand how to get the most out of their time in the gym. This section is about just that and if you follow the simple steps here you will find that you get further than just blindly going into a gym and lifting weights.

Always determine what is most important during this training session. What is the most important exercise you will perform today? If you are training chest, the answer would likely be the bench press. If you plan to work legs, the most important thing you can do is squat. You should begin each workout with whatever is most crucial to your progress. Hitting the heaviest lift first will allow you to expend the most energy on it and thus make the most gains.

Group together like exercises. What this means is that if your workout consists of 3 chest exercises and 4 biceps exercises, perform the 3 chest exercises consecutively and do the same for the biceps. If you allow you muscles to rest while you work another muscle then you are not working as intensely as possible. Training is all about having the highest intensity possible while avoiding injury and overtraining, so use this knowledge to your advantage.

Do not skip leg day. For that matter, do not skip any muscle group. If you plan on being a bodybuilder you should understand that you are only as strong as your weakest link. If you have a well-developed upper body but have never trained your legs then this is a glaring flaw in your physique. Take the time to hit each individual muscle and you will be grateful that you did.

Rest an adequate amount in between sets. The general consensus is that about 60 to 90 seconds is enough rest, any less and you will not have enough energy to perform as you should while taking a longer rest will decrease the intensity of the workout. Many people disregard this and talk in between sets for upwards to 5 minutes but in the long run this will only harm you.

Form

Although it is commonly thrown out of the window, form is mandatory if you wish to avoid injury and perform exercises as they were intended. Form refers to the movement used during an exercise, while proper form refers to performing this movement correctly and poor form refers to incorrectly performing an exercise.

To better understand this I will give an example in the form of a pull-up. When performing a pull-up your legs should remain stationary and your body should only move up and down, this is proper form. If you allow your legs to move and swing while pulling yourself up then you are using poor form. In this example using poor form leads to an ineffective exercise, but in most cases poor form will quickly lead to injury. Always make sure that you understand proper form for each exercise and ensure that you are performing it in this manner before adding heavy weight.

Cardio

Cardio is a debated subject among bodybuilders. Some believe it is the best thing ever while some hate it due to the fact that it burns calories (and as you get bigger you need to consume a significant amount of calories to maintain that weight). My personal opinion is that cardio should be at least a small part of your training regimen, if only for the health benefits for your heart.

As a bodybuilder, since you do not want to burn unnecessary calories, I advise you to implement a cardio exercise that kills two birds with one stone. For example, if you run sprints up a hill then you are getting a cardio workout as well as training your legs. If running is not your thing then you can hit a heavy bag. Boxing will help develop your upper body and is also a good method of self-defense. The point is to get creative and do something that will make the loss of calories worth it.

Training Splits

The way that you try will vary drastically based on how often you plan on going to the gym. Can you only go 3 days a week? Then each session will likely be longer and more intense than if you can make it 5 days a week. This is not a suggestion but rather a rule. If you try to train as intensely 5 times a week as you would if you were only going 3 times then you will end up overtraining and becoming injured.

Once you decide on how many times per week you are going you will need to decide how to divide the days up so that you work each muscle during the week. A common split is upper/lower body and this is what I currently do. For example, say that you plan on going to the gym 4 days a week. Monday and Thursday you can work upper body while Tuesday and Friday you can work lower body. Using this split allows you to have sufficient rest time during the week (you get the weekend and Wednesday as rest days) and also gives you two days a week for each muscle group.

If you have 5 days a week you can divide the muscles even further, and if you only have 2 days then you will likely have to perform full body workouts on both days. You get the point, it can change based on your needs. The main points to keep in mind are that you work each muscle about twice a week and you give it ample time to heal in between those two workouts. Aside from that you can change it to fit your personal schedule.

Plateaus

After years or even months of training it is common to hit a plateau. This is basically a wall in the way of your progress. Plateauing can occur for any number of reasons but there is usually a way around it.

First you must examine your current training regimen. How long has it been that you have been performing the same exercise on the same days of the week with the same weight? You should always be increasing intensity in some way so if your workout stays the same for too long you will not make progress. Most people fix this by routinely raising the weight on each exercise when possible, however eventually even this will not be enough.

When you find that you are not becoming stronger at a particular exercise it is possible that your body needs a change. Find a new, but similar, exercise that works the same muscle. Perform this for several weeks or months until you stop progressing at it and move back to the old exercise and you will likely find that you can begin progressing at it again.

If changing things up does not work then you should try taking a short break from training altogether. A week off will allow your body to recuperate and might be all that you need to break through your plateau.

Injury

Injury is a serious concern in all sports and weight lifting is no exception. The constant pressure of heavy weight on the bone and joints can seriously harm your body. Although it is possible that you will become injured at some point in your career no matter what, you can greatly reduce the chances of this by following proper precautions.

First and foremost, use proper form. Time and time again lifters assume that form is something that they can ignore which always leads to an injury. Improper form puts unnecessary stress on your body and will almost definitely lead to harm either now or down the road. If you are not sure if your form is what it needs to be then ask a trainer or other experienced lifter to critique you until you are confident that everything is as it should be.

The next step to avoiding injury is listening to your body. Over time you will be able to tell the difference between good pain and bad pain. Good pain is the burn that you feel during an exercise telling you that progress is being made. Bad pain is felt in the bone or joints, a stinging or snapping sensation. This is usually a precursor to a more serious injury and you should have a sports doctor take a look at it before it worsens. I say a sports doctor because a general doctor will not know exactly what is going on and will most likely tell you to stop whatever is causing the pain. On the other hand, a doctor that has seen many sports related injuries will have experience with whatever is ailing you and will likely be able to make a more detailed diagnosis.

A common cause of injury among weight lifters is not working supporting muscles. You need to realize that, for example, while your biceps might be strong enough to curl a certain weight your forearms may not have the strength to support the lift. This is true for any compound lift. You should always work supporting muscles just as you would primary muscles. Not only will it prevent injury but it is required for a well-rounded physique.

Recovery

If you maintain a balanced diet, train with the appropriate intensity, and still are not seeing progress then this means that you are not allowing yourself enough time to recover. There can always be too much of a good thing and this applies to bodybuilding as well. Overtraining is a term used to describe when someone frequently trains the same muscle without allowing it time to repair. Although you might think you are gaining an advantage by training day in and day out, the reality is that you are doing more harm than good.

Rest days are in used to prevent overtraining. Although you are not actually training, these days are just as important as days in the gym as this is when you become stronger. When you are training your muscle fibers become damaged and unable to lift the weight after a certain amount of reps. This causes your body to tell these muscles to grow back stronger in order to deal with this heavy weight, and this process occurs during sleep and rest days.

Many lifters do not realize that in addition to rest days they also must get adequate sleep each night. This is ideally 8 hours but at least 7 if you would like to make progress as fast as possible. The reasoning is the same behind why rest days are necessary, hours spent sleeping repair the body and gives it time to prepare for the next training session.

After an intense workout you will feel tired but you most likely will not feel sore until the next morning. This is known as DOMS (Delayed Onset Muscle Soreness). As a beginner all you really need to know is that this is a good sign. Soreness means that your muscles were damaged and are now repairing and becoming stronger. As time goes on you may not experience DOMS and this is normal. Just because you are not does not mean you did not have an intense workout your body is simply becoming adjusted to the sensation.

Gym Etiquette

No beginner's guide should leave out such an important topic as etiquette, and yet I have not once seen this subject officially covered. I am going to do you and everyone else at the gym a favor and go over a few basics of how to behave and common mistakes to avoid.

The fault with most beginners is that they are not serious about weight lifting. They go to the gym with a group of friends, socialize, text for several minutes after sets, and generally tie up the equipment. This is a waste of your time as well as anyone waiting on whatever you happen to be using. Nothing is more irritating than being halfway into your workout, adrenaline flowing, and having to wait for a bench because someone is sitting and texting for 10 or 20 minutes. If you absolutely need to talk to someone while at the gym make sure that you get off of the bench or machine that you are at so others can use it while you are busy.

You may have heard the phrase "Do not curl in the squat rack" already and this is such a huge mistake that new lifters make, but it goes further than curling. In most gyms there is only a few squats racks in the entire area and this is the only possible area that you can safely perform squats. You can curl, deadlift, military press, or do whatever else you want anywhere in the gym so leave the squat rack open for squatters.

If you have the strength to use a weight, you should have the strength to put it back on the rack. Unfortunately, many people think it is fine to leave piles of dumbbells on the floor and to leave a bar with various plates stacked on it. Do not be one of these people. Take the extra minute to pick the weights up and I promise you will save yourself and everyone else a good deal of annoyance.

The more experienced you come, the more opportunities you have to share that experience. It is common courtesy to help out someone if you see them using poor form, but do not be rude about it. This extends beyond form, once you are an experienced bodybuilder you are likely to have a lot of advice that can help beginners and you should share any knowledge that you have when given the opportunity.

Choosing a Gym

Now that you know how to train effectively it is time to decide on a gym. Since it is likely that you will be spending a lot of time here you should put a decent amount of thought into your decision. First, consider what is most important to you as a weightlifter. Are you interested in a gym that is open 24/7 or do you care more about a large variation of equipment? Perhaps it is important to you that you do not have to wait long for a machine or a bench, in which case you should make sure the gym you are considering is not overcrowded during the time you plan to workout.

The gym itself is not the only thing you need to take into consideration. Distance from your home should also be taken into account. Remember that you will be making this trip several times a week and it should be convenient for you to get there. Price is another factor, if you are on a budget then it might make more sense to get a membership at a less than ideal gym and save the extra cash.

If a traditional gym does not suit your needs then there is another option: building a home gym. This can be beneficial for a number of reasons. Over an extended time period of several years a home gym might be less expensive than a continuous membership to a gym. You also get the bonus of having no wait time to use any of the equipment and you do not even have to travel to get there.

There are several ways to go about building a home gym if you decide to go this route. The more expensive option would be to build a small building near your home and buy all of the equipment you might possibly need for your lifting career at once. This could potentially save you money by buying weights in a set (this is cheaper than buying them individually) but you might not get any use out of them for quite some time. If you would prefer a cheaper choice, you can empty out a room in your house and buy any weights that you are currently using in your workouts. As you get stronger you can buy new weights which means you will never buy anything that you are not going to be using in the near future however over time this could be more expensive. It is important to note that if you build a small gym you can always invite friends and family to exercise there for a much cheaper fee that they would be charged at a traditional gym and in this way you could earn back some of the money you invested (and maybe even make a profit).

Regardless which path you go with, choose a gym that will allow you get the most out of the time you will be investing there.

Choosing a Partner

One component of training that many people overlook is the value of a good partner. With the right person at your side you can make sure that every session is worth the time you put into it. However, you should understand that the reverse is also true. If you decide to choose a bad partner then you will waste time and effort in the gym.

So, what is the best way to go about choosing a gym partner? Whoever you choose should have the same goals as you and ideally be farther ahead in their bodybuilding career than you are. If your fellow lifter already has more experience than you then that means that you will be able to go to this person for advice. Direct advice from another weight lifter is invaluable as questions *constantly* come up that can be easily answered by someone with practical knowledge.

While it is simply beneficial that your partner be more experienced than you I believe it should be mandatory that he or she have the same goal as you. If your goals differ (one of you is a powerlifter and the other a bodybuilder) then your training style will be different and your schedule may be different, it just is not as helpful as if you have someone working towards the same end result you are.

The final consideration in deciding on a partner is taking into account their level of dedication. If you go with someone who skips a workout more often than not then they have no real value to you as a partner. Even if they never skip a session, make sure that whoever you choose to go with is not wasting time in the gym goofing off or having lengthy conversations. Socializing can be done at any other time, the hours you put into a workout should be spent solely on pushing your body to its limits.

Although I think it is best that everyone find a partner to workout with, going solo is a perfectly viable option. Depending on your personality you might even be more effective training alone. The pros to this are obvious: less wait time in between sets, you can complete a workout faster, and your schedule will not rely on anyone else. This choice also comes with a pretty heavy drawback though. If you train alone, there is nobody there to push you to finish your set. Where you might drive yourself to finish and compete if you had a partner you might simply give up and quit if you are on your own. As you become more experienced you will learn whether you work best alone or as part of a group, but whatever you choose make sure that your decision will allow you to get the most out of your training.

Scheduling

A common excuse that I hear time and time again is "I am too busy to fit in a workout". Very rarely is this actually the case. Do you have time to watch an hour of television or more a day? Could you stand to wake up a little earlier each day? Are there 3 or more days out of the week that you do not work? You get where I am going with this. Regardless of your schedule, you can make time to train.

Usually it is rather easy to make time for a workout. Many modern companies have a gym available for employees, in which case you can go on your lunch break or immediately after your shift ends. Otherwise it is a simple matter of either finding an hour during the day where you are not busy or waking up early enough to train before you need to get ready for the day.

For the most part it does not make much of a difference when you train. Many people like to do it first thing in the morning as they claim this is when they have the most energy and it helps them to wake up, but it really boils down to personal preference. If you decide to train before bed, however, it should be noted that if you exercise too late you might have difficulty falling asleep.

I have mentioned several times that you need about an hour to train. This is because in most cases you will want this length of time set aside for a session. However, based on your training split, you might need less or more time depending on the intensity level that you are going for with each session. If you plan to exercise 5 days a week then you will need less time per day than if you are only going to the gym 3 days a week. Follow these general rules and you will be fine. This guide is based around beginners and if you are a beginner then the most important thing is to train when you can make time.

Common Terms

Macros – This is short for macronutrients, a type of food (e.g., fat, protein, carbohydrate) required in large amounts in the human diet

PR – Personal record

Rep – Short for repetition, this is one full movement of an exercise. For example, during bench press a repetition is the movement from starting position down to your chest back to starting position.

Set – A set is several consecutive reps performed without taking a rest in between. If you perform 10 consecutive curls without a break then that is 1 set of 10.

Additional Resources

supplementreviews.com – As the name implies, this website is my source for reviews of any supplement that I would possibly like to purchase. It has a category for any supplement you can think of as well as reviews from real lifters. Products are rater on everything from effectiveness to how suspicious the company selling it seems. Through careful research on this site you will know whether a supplement is legit or a scam and whether it will give you the results you want or not. If you are the type of person that likes to review products you can also create your own account and let other potential buyers know about your experience with the supplement.

bodybuilding.com – Again, self-explanatory, but this website is a great place for all things bodybuilding. Exercises can be searched and you will get a video showing how to perform them with proper form along with detailing which muscles it builds. The forums have hundreds of bodybuilders that you can ask for specific advice or look to for motivation. There is even a section called "bodyspace" where you can upload progress pictures and receive comments on your progress.

www.ingramcontent.com/pod-product-compliance
Lightning Source LLC
Chambersburg PA
CBHW061933280526
45787CB00004B/1590